A Mother's Guide to Self- Reliant Health Care

To Melanie Renae

The girl with wisdom well beyond her years

Any sources that I name are ones I actually use. I am not affiliated with any of these companies (with the exception of do Terra©) in any financial way. Colonial Bloom® is my own creation. My opinions are my own from my own experience.

Many of the remedies in this book are available on my website www.colonialbloom.com for purchase if you are not ready to make your own.

However, the purpose of this book is to teach self-reliance. My hope is you will make your own when you are ready.

Preface: Why I Do What I Do

Every mother has a journey she has been through that teaches her the best way to care for her children. Mine has been one fraught with everything from carnival ride happiness to terror on the high seas. From "It worked!!!" to "What can I possibly do for this?" There have been times when a doctor of conventional medicine has saved my bacon. There have also been several times I have come home from that same office more frustrated than when I went in. This little book is a guide to help mothers who may need a spring board to care for their families in a more natural way. There is **no *shame*** in having to go to the Doctor, but there is ***great satisfaction*** in caring for your own when possible without professional medical help.

My name on the cover page is followed by the initials M.O.M This is a self-claimed title. It means Master of Much. Every mother has to be that for her family. When a mother is the master of her family's health, it brings great joy.

My journey began when my first-born child came to Earth. We were so excited and exhausted. He began crying all the time, was fussy, had a fever. I didn't know what to do. I took him in to our family doctor and lo and behold – he had an ear infection. I gladly went to the pharmacy to pick up the prescription. Within a week we were done with the medicine and life was so good again. Well, this scenario happened seven more times within his *first nine months* of life. It was exhausting! Our doctor suggested we put ventilation tubes in his ears – I was ready to try anything. These tubes helped the infections to stop, but lead to another list of issues with hearing problems.

A few years later I was talking to a friend when my second child had an ear infection. She told me of a chiropractor who had suggested a vodka and vinegar combination to put in the ear. It worked for her. I was willing to try anything to avoid what we had been through. It sounded a little weird, but hey, why not?

I followed the instructions (found here in the ear chapter) and it worked. I have not used antibiotics for ear infections since. Here's the thing, antibiotics (they have their place don't get me wrong) kill all bacteria in the body. There are **good** bacteria that die in the intestines that die in vain! They shouldn't have to go. They are the good guys. They are needed for proper digestion (which will be discussed later). It makes better sense to kill only the offending bacteria if at all possible. The ear happens to be one of those places.

When you are self-reliant with the healthcare of your family, you don't have to worry about dragging your kid to a place that makes you wonder if they will be coming out with something worse than that which you are taking them in. Who sat in the chair you are sitting in? What did they have? In your home, you know who has been there. You know when the toilet or sink was cleaned last. You have better control of the environment in your home. There is peace of mind with that.

This guide is for the normal, everyday illnesses that seem to be the rite of passage for parenting. If you are looking for help with a specific serious illness (cancer, diabetes, etc) you may not find much for these issues in this book. My prayers are with you.

Because I am not a licensed physician, I can't tell you what to do, but I can tell you what I do. Decide for yourself if the information is what you choose to do with your own family.

I love helping people realize the power they have to care for their families in a less expensive, less stressful way. Let us begin…

Chapter 1

GET YOUR OWN ROCKS MAHONRI!

I believe most people would agree that a book is only as good as the experience and knowledge that the author has to offer. I could write a book about mechanical engineering, but it wouldn't be very good because I do not have the experience or schooling to make it a very useful book. However, when it comes to self-reliant health care I have a lot of experience because I am a mother. Be aware that my experiences are not your experiences. Step one to being self-reliant is to find answers for yourself.

In the Book of Mormon, we meet Jared and his brother Mahonri. The Lord had given direction to cross the ocean. They were not ship builders. The ships they were instructed to build were different than they had ever seen before. No one knew how to light the ships. Mahonri inquired of the Lord. The Lord basically said, "Do a little research, think about it and then tell me how you would like my help."

Many times when I have found things that work for me or my family, others will ask me what to do for their family. It isn't that I do not want to share my knowledge, because I do- but sometimes you have to do your own research to figure out what will work for you.

My number one tool as a mother is prayer. There are many, many times that I didn't know what else to do. All advice and medicine were not working. I needed to find another way. Prayers are answered; sometimes we have to be patient.

To illustrate this, I am going to use a few examples. This story is one of my favorites in all of LDS church history.

Amanda Barnes Smith was the mother of a child named Alma who was severely wounded at the Haun's Mill Massacre. His hip was in such bad shape that none of the bones were together.

With her son Willard by her side they prayed together for help and inspiration. She told Alma " The Lord has made it known to me that He will make you well, but you must lie on your stomach for a few weeks." She then took white ashes from the camp fire to make a weak lye and washed the wound. Then she made a poultice of slippery elm tree roots. When the poultice turned black, the wound was washed again and the poultice was changed. He fully recovered.

This story is one that I was not familiar with, but when I read it, I gained even more respect for Lucy Mack Smith. She is one of my heroes. When Sister Smith saw that her daughter Sophronia who had typhus (which is kind of like mono with rashes, high fever and ache) looked very close to death. A doctor had been helping her for 89 days. He told her there was nothing else he could do. She and her husband knelt by their bedside and prayed that Sophronia would be spared a little longer. Sister Smith picked up her frail daughter, wrapped her in a blanket and began pacing the floor. Some who were there tried to tell her that it was no use and to just accept that she was going to die. However, Lucy did not give up. Sophronia began to sob and from that time forward began to recover. You will not find that "cure" in any medical journal.

So, I guess that the bottom line is with prayer, a little research and the willingness to roll up your sleeves and get to work, a mother can be empowered beyond belief. **With that being said I hope you enjoy the ideas, tips and tricks that I have learned to help you on your own journey.**

Chapter 2

Prevention The Best Medicine

One of my heroes, Benjamin Franklin said: "An ounce of prevention is worth a pound of cure." I couldn't agree more!

There are many conspiring political reasons that some things are added to our food or products we use to keep us healthy and happy. I won't be discussing those even though they exist. I will merely be highlighting some of these dangerous ingredients and why they should be avoided.

When I first began to research these additives and what they could do to the body, I was overwhelmed and frustrated. It seemed there were so many things to avoid. Then I realized that "by small and simple things are great things brought to pass." (Alma 37:33) Less is more. Stick with Mother Nature, she knows what she's doing.

I love herbs! I love what they do to balance the body. However, it would be better not to have to break them out if there were a way to avoid the problem in the first place. Just remember "line upon line" – it might take a while to cut these ingredients out, but it can be done. Here are a few suggestions for the BEST medicine:

1. Do Read Labels on Food: I have done a lot of label reading. Labels can mean the difference between healthy or not healthy. Avoid things in your family's diet with these things:

MSG – it can cause headaches and colic for nursing babies. It is found in soups, boullion, premade meals (like Hamburger Helper etc), and so much more!

Aspartame – this artificial sugar is toxic. It is a neuro-toxin and can cause headaches, blindness and a list of other things with constant consumption. It is a chemical and not close to nature

AT ALL. It is better to have refined white highly processed sugar… seriously.

Propylene glycol – This is added to commercial coconut. It is basically antifreeze. This also found in lotions, some deodorants and baby diaper cream. It has been linked to fertility problems. So, why put it in a diaper cream?

High Fructose Corn Syrup – This sounds safe enough; it is made out of corn right? Well, it is processed so much that the pancreas doesn't know what in the world it is. It is really hard for the pancreas to metabolize which can lead to blood sugar issues. This can be found in everything from Katsup, to breakfast cereal to soda. Because of consumer demands, manufacturers are beginning to change from this syrup back to sugar without any compromise to the flavor.

Vegetable Shortening and Margarine – These are also highly processed fats and the body can't function properly when they are consumed.

Aluminum – This is added to baking powder. Aluminum is a heavy metal that has been linked to neurological disorders. Aluminum free baking powder is usually found next to the canisters that do have it. All aluminum (and Teflon/non stick) cooking pans should be taken to the thrift store. Cook with stainless steel or cast iron.

If You Can't Pronounce It – Look It Up – I could go on and on about chemicals added to our food for preservation and flavor, but the bottom line is, if you don't know what it is, do a little research. This is a huge reason to preserve your own food stuffs from your own garden.

2. <u>Do</u> Read Labels on Skin and Oral Care Items:

SLS or Sodium Laurel Sulfate (i.e. Laureth) – This chemical is a synthetic version of coconut oil used as a surfactant (i.e. to clean out the oil and make it bubble like crazy). It is linked to skin issues like eczema. There are several "natural" manufacturers that have their products available on the internet and many health food stores. They make SLS free shampoos and tooth paste. Just remember to read the label.

Fluoride – Dental journals for years have gone back and forth regarding the safety of fluoride. I say, "If you can't make up your mind, just keep it out!" Some types of fluoride do occur naturally, but constant exposure to any fluoride eventually leads to bone decay. Some fluoride is a byproduct of aluminum processing which is very toxic. Health food stores carry fluoride free, but just to make sure, read the label. Some companies tout "natural" when they are just as far from it as the big commercial guys.

Aspartame – Again, this is used to flavor chewing gum and toothpaste labeled as "sugar free". Look for toothpaste flavored with Xylitol instead. Xylitol also doesn't have a synthetic aftertaste like Aspartame.

Parabens – These guys are a family of preservatives for lotions and other skin care products. The first names are "Methal" and "Propal". They have been linked to all kinds of health issues. There are lotions available that are preserved with natural alcohols that work great and are paraben free

If You Can't Pronounce It – Look It Up – Health and Beauty manufacturers are required to list any natural ingredients by their Latin names…we all speak Latin so that makes all kinds of sense. Because of this, everything on a bottle sounds bad. For instance if I said "tocopheryl acetate", you might ask me to watch my language. In reality I am talking about vitamin E.

This is also used as a preservative, but is natural. If you have any questions, look it up. If it is synthetic avoid it.

3. Do Choose a Healthy Lifestyle:

The Word of Wisdom is to be used as a guide to keep our bodies healthy. If I wanted to eat a healthy diet, there are so many conflicting ideas and diet plans. Where do I get the proper information? I am sure someone would disagree with my interpretation, but here is my opinion.

If I were to eat meat sparingly, what exactly does that mean? Sparingly is to spare the animal. Sparingly doesn't specifically say "become a vegetarian" but it also doesn't say "steak and eggs every night honey!!" either. In the latter days there are so many bad manufacturing practices like radiating meats to kill bacteria (sounds really safe right?) that in all honesty we need to make it a matter of prayer. We pray over our food and there is a reason for that.

Some things aren't specific in the Word of Wisdom and we need to use our own judgment. Listen to the Spirit and look to sources that use sound practices for education. "Organics" are a good choice, but again, there are still conspiring things that happen in the "organic" world. Here are a few things I have learned:

Fruit should be eaten alone – if it is mixed with grain or protein, it can ferment in the body and instead of being healthy for you, can actually contribute to health issues. Sure, you can have that peach cobbler, but make it more rare than the norm.

Eat As Many Fresh Foods As You Can: Enzymes are our digestive system's best friend. They help us digest our food. Heavenly Father created food to carry its own enzymes to aid in the digestion of that food. If we eat too many enzyme depleted or deficient food from processing and heat, we begin to see digestive issues. Some of these issues can be, IBS (irritable bowel syndrome), gas, constipation, etc. Live foods equals happy bowels. Enzyme supplements can also be found at health food stores or online. If your fresh foods and vegetables must be cooked, try to do it at the lowest possible temperatures to keep those enzymes alive. If they are boiled, all enzymes have died.

Sweets Thing: I am the last person on the earth to tell you to not eat sugar. I love chocolate, cakes, cookies etc. However; there are so many studies that suggest that sugar is a poison and can lead to attention issues and glycemic issues, that I should probably address it. Even the touted "more healthy" sugars like xylitol (made from birch trees), agave and even honey will still mess with your blood sugar numbers. The bottom line is: moderation. If you must have something sweet, have sugar, do not go for the aspartame or any of the artificial sugars. Stevia is the only sweetener that I know of that does not make sugar numbers spike. The closer to nature the stevia is, the better. The more processed (like white powder from a green plant is not natural) you find, the less benefits you get from it. Stevia also kills yeast! Xylitol inhibits the growth of yeast. Yeast overgrowth is not our friend (i.e. UTIs, athlete's foot, vaginal yeast infections, thrush, etc.)

Drink Water, Not Soda – Okay, so we reach one of those "this isn't specifically mentioned in the Word of Wisdom" things. If you take the basic components of soda, it becomes a no brainer for your health. The sugar content is about half of the silly drink. The carbonation is carbon dioxide, the waste product from our breathing. It also dehydrates the body instead of becoming a "refreshing beverage". Diet sodas have aspartame as the sweetener which is even worse than the regular high sugar content. The caffeine becomes addictive and can be a wooleybooger to get off of. Some withdrawal symptoms can be headaches, insomnia, depression, irritability and even flu like symptoms. You would think we were talking about the hard stuff. Soda once in a while is okay I guess, but you can see how a 44 ouncer three times a day can adversely affect your health and break down your immune system, your muscles, and dehydrate you. A word on "energy drinks"- wow, these are really bad for your health! There are teenage kids who have been admitted to the hospital because of irregular heart function. The caffeine content is so high that the heart gets off its regular pattern. There was even a young girl who already had heart problems and drank them anyway. She had a heart attack and died. Caffeine puts your adrenal glands on a high, when it comes down the adrenal gland is exhausted. Consumers think, "Man, I have no energy today, I need another energy drink." When the adrenal gland is spent – another energy drink isn't going to help it repair. You can't put a fire out with more gasoline. Do your body a favor and never drink these.

Water on the other hand cleans and hydrates the cell. With more than half of the body made of water, it just makes sense to refill it with clean water. If you squeeze a little lemon in your water…ahhh now that's refreshing. Fruit juices have been so highly processed that the true vitamins no longer exist so they have to add them. They are mostly sugar. Because of the processing, in order for the body to process fruit juices, it will remove calcium from your bones to assimilate it. If you want fruit juice, make your own. It carries the active enzymes and tastes way better.

Another note on water: It is becoming more and more apparent that water tainted with lots of chlorine and fluoride (among other things in some cities) does not clean the cells as water was intended to. These chemicals can adversely affect the heart and bones. There are house filtration systems (not reverse osmosis) that clean the water and make it usable once again for the body. These filtration systems can be expensive, but not as expensive as hospital bills. If nothing else, get a filter for the water you drink. Be sure to change the filters as often as the manufacturer suggests. Bottled water isn't necessarily the best option either. It is expensive and the water isn't that much more "pure" than filtered water, no matter where they claim which mountain spring in the Himalayas they got it from.

A Note on Allergies: We face many challenges despite modern technology where we are seeing a decline in health instead of improvement. One of those is the HUGE rise in allergies to so many different foods. The human race is having reactions to everything from eggs to wheat and corn and dairy…the list goes on and on. We are seeing this because of the generations of processed foods. The more we process, the more the body is saying "STOP IT!!! GET BACK TO BASICS!" Allergies can be something that can make a mother cry harder than just about anything else that I know of. It can exhaust every energy of her soul. DON'T GIVE UP! I have known families who have received acupuncture and the allergy went away. There are special diets such as GAPS that can put the body back on track and balance it again.

What's That Smell?: You know when you walk into somebody's home and they have one of those plug in air fresheners? It smells nice, but oh boy those scents are anything but good for you. They have phthalates that are linked to various respiratory problems. The smells of home are smells we remember all our lives. Studies have been done linking the sense of smell to activate the memory part of the brain more than any other sense. If you must have something pretty, find an essential oil you enjoy and have it diffused into the air. It is much better for you and they are real smells, not fake ones. I like to make a nice homemade potpourri by slicing up some oranges and putting them in a pot of warmed apple juice. Add a touch of cinnamon and clove - put it on low all day. Not only that, by the end of the day you have a nice wassail to drink!

Wash Those Hands: Never underestimate the power of a good hand washing! There were times that I really didn't think that washing hands made a difference…I know, back in the days when I was really naïve. Then I began to see the pattern. We would go to the store, and almost like clockwork, within one or two days somebody would be sick. This happened the most in the winter time. Now, before they are allowed to eat any treat we get from the store, the rule is we have to wash our hands first. That has made a big difference in how often we get sick. Another thing that I try to do (especially in the winter) is to find carts at the store that have been out in the sun for a while. The sun is way better at disinfecting than those wipes full of chemicals. Those chemicals can make the immune system weak. Also, don't use "antibacterial" soaps. They can also make the immune system weak. Just plain soap and warm water gets the job done.

And the Winner IS! : I think the **number one** thing that has made a huge difference in our family's ability prevent disease is by not consuming fresh (raw or store-bought) cow's milk. Does that sound crazy? I had read in books and online that the best way to consume was by eating only cultured dairy. "Cultured" means cultures added to it. Yogurt, kefir, and cheese are examples of this. In the sources I had read, they said that the protein in cow's milk (called casein) is too hard for the human body to digest on its own. When enzymes are added to it, they are better digested. I brushed that information aside. I have to have my milk! I've been raised on raw cow's milk most of my life – I couldn't live without it. Winter after winter we would pass around the same germs and just fight it the entire season. Then there was a class I attended that changed my life. The teacher mentioned this one more time and for some reason it clicked. So, our family went cold turkey off of cow's milk. We began drinking rice milk. I had a few complaints for a week or so. I wasn't sure I was going to be able to keep it up because my job as a mother is to keep the peace. But I stuck to my guns, and lo and behold, that first winter was AMAZING! We had a cough or two, but that was IT! The entire winter I kept shaking my head saying, "It must be a fluke! There is no way that we haven't gotten sick." But for the second winter in a row (at the

14

time of this publication), we have again had success. We have had a little bit of sickness, but we aren't passing it to each other over and over like we were before. There are other kinds of alternative milks like almond, cashew and coconut if you prefer a different flavor than rice. Avoid soy though, because of the estrogen hormones that are naturally occurring. They cause issues in males and females. The best part is these alternative milks can be made in your kitchen. Some may say, "Well, what about your calcium? If you want strong bones, you need to drink milk." Well, a friend pointed this out to me and I will never forget it! She said "Where do cows get their calcium?" "Uh, I don't know." I replied. "They get it from green food," she said. "Oh, duh," said I. So, the bottom line is, eat fresh green food daily.

Chapter 3

The Herbal Toolbox

Heavenly Father has granted more than one way to help us provide for our healthcare needs through nature. I will be highlighting a few of those in this chapter.

The philosopher Hippocrates is credited with saying: "Let food be thy medicine, and let medicine be thy food." If there is anything I would agree with a guy who walked around wearing his bed sheet, this would be it! In fact, I think he is smarter than many of the supposed geniuses of today by this quote alone.

There are a few glimpses of references to herbs in the scriptures. There is one found in Alma 46:40 that says:

"And there were some who died with fevers, which at some seasons of the year were very frequent in the land – but not so much with fevers, because of the excellent qualities of the many plants and roots which God had prepared to remove the cause of diseases, to which men were subject by the nature of the climate."

There is also a verse in Doctrine and Covenants 89 (where the Word of Wisdom is found) that says:

"Every herb in the season thereof, and every fruit in the season thereof; all of these to be used with prudence and thanksgiving."

What is prudence? It means "before you throw any herb at something, do a little research first." There are so many sources for finding what types of herbs are "prudent" for what type of ailment.

In verse 8, it says that tobacco is not for the "body" or the "belly" but it is to be used for bruises and sick cattle. Not all herbs are good to be taken internally.

Herbs to Know

Here is a list of my favorite herbs and roots. These are the herbs that I would purchase and have on hand. (Be sure to check out the sources chapter to find quality places to find these)

Cayenne	Licorice root	Sage
Chaparral (aka creosote)	Mullein	Yarrow
Comfrey	Oregon Grape root	Yerba Santa
Elder Flower	Osha Root	Yellow dock
Ginger	Peppermint	Wild Tobacco
Goldenseal	Rosemary	

Foods to Know

These are regular foods that are EXCELLENT for keeping you healthy and help you heal. These are a great idea to have on hand.

Lemon juice	Aloe vera gel (the pure leaf, not the green stuff found in the sun screen isle)
Garlic	Honey (raw – uncooked/unpasteurized if possible)

Essential Oils to Know

Lately there has been a big boom with essential oils. Good quality oils are the ones you want to use. Companies make different profit margins by how the plants for the oils are grown, harvested and processed. I have sources listed where I get the oils I use. Those sources are listed in the "Sources" section of this book.

Peppermint	Lemon	Lavender
Clary Sage	Oregano	Melaleuca

Spices in the Cupboard to Know

Sage	Ginger Powder	Cinnamon
Clove	Turmeric	Cayenne

You may be surprised at the spices in your cupboard that also have medicinal properties. That brings new meaning to "Let food be thy medicine, and let medicine be thy food."

Extras to Know

Bentonite Clay is one of my favorite tools. It is a magnetic clay that literally draws impurities from the skin. I have seen small miracles from acne clearing up to vanishing bruises using this awesome stuff ! It is best to purchase the powder that has an infinite shelf life because it is clay. When you're ready to use it, add water a little at a time until you get a clay like consistency then apply. I will explain how I use it in later chapters.

Colloidal Silver is also a favorite tool. Back many years ago in the pioneer days, I have read reports of those wise pioneers putting a silver coin in their bucket of milk to keep it from spoiling. Silver inhibits bacterial growth and kills it. It however doesn't kill "all" bad bacteria, but I do use it a lot. C-Silver got a bad rap a few years ago when a man appeared on a popular midday show who was blue. He was blaming his discoloration on Colloidal Silver. First, he took way too much; he was drinking several glasses a day. Second he was taking it all the time – that is way too much. C-Silver is best used in ½ teaspoon every half hour or so. It does work very well. Moderation is still the key.

Chapter 4

Ways to Use Herbs

There are a number of different ways to use herbs. There are some I prefer over others, but this preference is based upon my experience and your preferences may be different.

Some would argue that the only ways that herbs can be used as described in the Word of Wisdom are as a poultice or compress because tea is a "hot drink". Additionally tinctures use alcohol to extract the medicinal properties and thus violate this commandment. Joseph Smith, after receiving the revelation, confirmed that "hot drink" was habit forming tea and coffee. Herbal teas are not habit forming. However, even herbal teas should be cooled before being consumed. In fact, a very useful herb has been named "Brigham Tea" or "Mormon Tea" because of its usefulness to the pioneers as they crossed the plains.

Doctrine and Covenants 89:7 says, "And again, strong drinks are not for the belly, but for the washing of your bodies." The most common way to make a tincture is through alcohol extraction. Vinegar and vegetable glycerin can also be used, but I believe using herbs this way is washing the body of microbials – internal and external. Neither vinegar nor vegetable glycerin tinctures have nearly the shelf life that alcohol does. This use of alcohol is in moderation because it is used by the dropper – not even a spoonful. That is way less alcohol than "Nyquil" or other over the counter cold and flu medicines.

My favorite place to purchase quality organic herbs is www.mountainroseherbs.com.

Tea	The crushed herb simply added to boiling water. The hot water extracts the goodies. Drink when cool.
Tincture	The herb is ground to a powder and added to a high quality alcohol for a period of time. When finished, the concoction is then strained. The extract is the liquid left over. If kept in a dark glass bottle in a dark cupboard, it will last for many years. Vanilla for cooking is made this way.
Poultice	The herb is crushed and then small amount of water is added to it and applied directly to the wound and left for a time. Sometimes poultices are left for hours or even days.
Compress	A bandage is soaked in a tea and then wrapped around the wound.

> ➤ Tea

Teas are easy, but they can be a little more time consuming than a tincture or poultice. Here is how I use teas:

- Bring a cup of water to a boil.
- Pour it into a mug with your tea bag in it
- Let it steep, usually about three minutes
- let it cool – add a little honey
- Drink

You can also make a gallon's worth and keep it in the fridge so that you don't have to keep making just a cup's worth.

This is how you can make a gallon of tea:

- Bring one gallon of water to boil
- Add one cup of crushed herb
- Let it steep 20-30 min

Strain out the leaves by pouring through a cheese cloth lined colander. Have a large bowl underneath to catch all the tea.

Put in a gallon container and put it in the fridge. It will stay good for about a week.

> **Tincture**

The way I prefer to take most herbs is by tincture. Tinctures are easy to make, they last a long time, and it is easier to give it to children than having them drink an entire cup of tea. The other benefit is that you don't have to boil a cup of water every time.

This is the way I use tinctures:

- Get a tiny cup (like a condiment cup or shot glass – tee hee) and put about three table spoons of water in it.
- Squirt one or two squirts of the tincture in the water
- Drink (some herbs are bitter, you may need to chase with a cup of water)

> **Poultice**

Poultices are awesome for things like bug bites, stings and open wounds. They are also good for all kinds of skin ailments and bruises. My favorite poultice is honey, cover disposable bandage with a plastic bag before applying the stretchy bandage (like an ace bandage) – otherwise it can get a bit messy.

This is how I use a poultice:

- Take about a table spoon of herb and mix with about half table spoon of water
- Apply to a disposable bandage (like gauze or even a paper towel)
- Put applied bandage over area
- Apply stretchy bandage (like an Ace bandage) to hold it in place

> **Compress**

As a mother, I don't really use compresses that much, but when I have used them, they have worked great. They work really well when you do not want little leaves from a poultice to get in a wound or rub in a burn.

This is how I use a compress:

- Make a tea
- Take a cotton muslin or linen bandage and soak it in the tea
- Wring it out, but keep slightly damp
- Lightly place on top of or wrap the wound

Chapter 5

Make Your Own "Get Better" Concoctions

I love using tinctures, and when I learned how to make them I was so excited! I won't call them "medicine" because I'm not a doctor, but they do help the person to "get better" so that's what I'll call them – "Get Better" concoctions.

There is more than one way to make these. We have already discussed what tinctures are made out of, but there are different ways to do that. These measurements are done by weight because volume can vary especially when we're talking about powdered herbs. All of the recipes in this section will require some tools.

- 1 pint glass jar with lid
- Cheese cloth or other fabric
- Small funnel
- 2 oz dark glass jar with dropper

Granny's Jug Ol' Fashioned Tincture

- 1 oz powdered herb
- 5 oz vodka

I like to take herbs that I have harvested or purchased and grind them in a coffee grinder. Take the powdered herb and put it in the pint glass jar. Add the alcohol. Swish it around to fully incorporate the two ingredients together. Put the lid on and put it in a dark cupboard. Shake it up once a day for two (for leaf herbs) or three (for root herbs) weeks. When the time is up, get your dark glass jar and put the funnel in the opening. Lay the fabric inside the funnel and spoon your concoction a little at a time into the cloth. Squeeze the extract out. Toss the left over herb in your compost pile. Repeat the spoon and squeeze method until it is all gone. What you have now is the power of nature in the form of an extract. These kinds of tinctures are good for 10 + years.

Vegetable glycerin tinctures are more suitable for younger children – say five and younger, or for those who just can't get over the alcohol thing. The vegetable glycerin is sweet so children are more likely to take it. The process is the same as the Ol' Fashioned kind, but with slight variation. These kind of tinctures are good for 1 to 2 years.

Vegetable Glycerin Tincture

- 1 oz powdered herb
- 2.5 oz food grade vegetable glycerin
- 2.5 oz water

Follow the same process as the Ol' Fashioned tincture. Tadah! You have your own alcohol free tincture!

The last way that you can make a tincture is to use vinegar. The process is basically the same. Don't use white vinegar. Find a raw apple cider vinegar with the mother in it (mother is the brown floaty stuff – looks weird, but is almost magical). Make sure your herbs are dried. These have the shelf life of one to two years, like the vegetable glycerin tinctures. Vinegar tinctures are going to have a stronger flavor.

Vinegar Tincture

1 oz dried herb

5 oz raw apple cider vinegar

Chapter 6

The Essentials of Oils

My first exposure to essential oils was not a positive one. I was invited to a gathering where a demonstration of how to use them would be done. When I got there, there was a feeling there that I wasn't comfortable with. It wasn't necessarily "hippie" or whatever, but I couldn't quite put my finger on it. To top it off, I ended up being the guinea pig and I smelled terrible for days. I swore I would never have ANYTHING to do with them ever again.

Well, thankfully, I have changed my tune. I use them almost on a daily basis now. What changed my mind? I had just had my third child and we were going on a walk as a family. It was summer time and the mosquitos were terrible! We stopped by a family friend's house to leave those obnoxious bugs outside for a bit. Before we left we told them how we had been breakfast, lunch, dinner, an afternoon snack and even "elevensies" to those pesky things. She said she had just the thing. She went to her cupboard and pulled out peppermint and lavender oils put them in a spray bottle with water and spritzed all of us. They didn't even get near us on the way home. I learned that night that not only can essential oils smell nice, but they are useful and it doesn't have to be a bad experience…in fact it can be a wonderful experience!!!

Within the last decade more information has become available on the uses of essential oils. In fact since the company "do Terra" has come out with their line of high quality essential oils, information and usage of essential oils by everyday people has just exploded! Sometimes oils of this quality can be out of range for many a bank account. My favorite website for organic quality oils is www.mountainroseherbs.com, - the price is reasonable and the quality is good.

The only problem that I have with using essential oils is that you can't go out into nature and harvest a bottle. But, if you do have it on hand, they last forever (if stored properly in a cool dark cupboard) and have many applications.

There are many books available that can do a better explanation on how to use them than I can, but I will share titles in the "sources" section of this book. I will tell you my experience because there is so much more to them than a chemical free bug repellant.

Most oils I use, I put one drop in a little water and down the hatch. Certain oils should not be taken internally. Other oils are best for their aromatic healing because the smells go right to the brain.

Note: Essential oils are exponentially stronger than tinctures. One drop will suffice the average usage.

Here are my favorites and what I use them for:

Peppermint	Tummy issues: overeating, gas, munchies A few drops on a wet washcloth makes a great dryer sheet Reduce fevers Add a few drops to brownies ☺ Invigorates the mind – helps wake you up!
Lemon	Tummy issues: flu like symptoms and settles stomach after throwing up.
Lavender	Calming Skin healing Bug repellant
Oregano	Anti- yeast Use a drop in Italian recipes Anti-bacterial

Melaleuca (or Tea Tree)	Anti-bacterial
Clary Sage	Sleep inducer, hormonal balancer
Rosemary	Helps rid bronchitis coughing Bacterial fever reducer
Eucalaptus	Coughs
Wintergreen	Coughs
Camphor	Coughs

There are so many more! Be sure to check Chapter 14 for my favorite book on how and which oils to use.

Chapter 7

Fevers

Fevers can be very scary, especially when it is a small child. In today's fast paced world, parents want the fever gone fast so they resort to medicines to do this. They have been taught that dehydration is eminent unless they give them these chemicals. Unfortunately, if given too frequently, these medicines can damage the liver.

True: You can dehydrate with a fever.

False: Getting rid of the fever gets rid of the sickness.

When you bring the fever down quickly, the body does not have a chance to do what it was designed to and raise the temperature to kill the germs that are attacking it. Fever reducing medicines make the body "yo-yo" with the temperature. It will come down and when the drugs wear off, the fever comes back up. When you let the fever give a constant heat to the germs you can kill more of them and recover faster. It may sound "mean" or "negligible" to let them have the fever for a while, but this helps the body naturally fight. Keeping hydrated is important. Sometimes children do not want to drink anything, which is where a lemonade popsicle can help. I'll give you a scenario-

Little Sally wakes up in the middle of night crying. She has a fever. It is 101.5 – that's hot, but not too hot. I draw a warm bath for Sally. The water is just above her 101.5 temperature. As the water cools it helps to bring the body temperature back in balance. I add about two table spoons of powdered ginger to the water. The ginger helps regulate the body heat. I only keep her in the tub as long as she is comfortable. I will help her drink some water to keep her hydrated. If she doesn't want to drink, I pull out a homemade lemonade popsicle (made with real lemon juice) that is sweet to help her get liquids.

I will usually let Sally have her fever for about 24 hours. If the fever does not come down on its own by then, it is time to help it along. If the infection is bacterial, (usually a low grade fever that gradually climbs up) I will give her some rosemary tincture every few hours. This will gradually bring the temperature back down. I will also give her either Oregon Grape Root tincture or Goldenseal Root tincture to help fight the bacteria.

If Sally has been throwing up or spiked a high fever out of nowhere, then it is probably viral. In my experience the only time bacteria makes a person throw up is if you suspect food poisoning:- like a ham and cheese sandwich that has been sitting in a hot car for a while…yeah, gross. If you think that the fever might be viral, then I would use elderflower tincture to bring down the fever. The lemon in the lemonade popsicle will also help to calm the stomach if vomiting is an issue.

Let's say I can't tell if it is viral or bacterial infection, you can give both rosemary and elderflower. The two combine just fine and it won't hurt a thing.

If a fever lasts more than a few days or is above 103° (which I've never seen), I suggest getting medical attention. There could be something else wrong.

Chapter 8

Tummy Aches and Throwey Uppies

One of the first times I remember receiving inspiration, I was in serious dire straits. Let me set the scene here for you. My oldest son woke me up at three in the morning, "Mom, my stomach doesn't…." Then he threw up on me in my bed. That was pleasant, let me tell you! Well, I cleaned him up, cleaned up my bed, cleaned everything in between. I tried to help him get comfortable again. A few hours later we went through the same thing. I finally had him sleep by the toilet. We did this for a few nights. When he was better, I was so excited!!! The next night, my second son came in and said, "Mom, my stomach doesn't…" Well, you get the idea. After he was better I was so excited! I could finally get some sleep! The next night my daughter came in and did the same routine. I was so exhausted. This was our routine for almost two weeks. When I thought we were in the clear, like clockwork, my oldest son came in at three in the morning. "Mom, my stomach doesn't feel…" I couldn't take anymore! Later that day I fell to my knees and just cried and prayed and told Him how I had done my best to be a good mom but it wasn't enough! What I was doing was not working. I asked Him to tell me what to do. The thought "lemon juice" came to my mind. What? Well, I haven't tried it so I'm going to give it a try. It was amazing!

I am not saying that lemon juice will cure all tummy ails, because that would be the wrong impression. It is funny, however, that the lessons we learn and remember the most is when we have to struggle for it. Then it means more to us. Please keep in mind that sometimes the body needs to vomit because it is trying to get rid of something.

The table below is a list of the things I have used for certain tummy issues.

What's wrong:	What to take:
I think I ate something that was bad	sage, licorice root, peppermint
My stomach just started hurting, I think I need to throw up	St. John's Wort, lemon juice, peppermint,
Something I ate is giving me gas and it hurts	enzymes, peppermint, lemon
My stomach is upset from the car ride	fennel, peppermint

Sometimes, no matter what you try, they still throw up. Small sips of lemon water (a teaspoon of lemon juice to 8 oz of water) and sucking on an ice cube will help keep them from getting dehydrated.

Sometimes there is an emotional reason for tummy upset. Sometimes it is anxiety, stress or sadness. In these cases a few drops of olive oil with a drop of lavender or clary sage oil rubbed on their feet can help them to relax.

I have one son who has a chronic upset stomach. He is allergic to going to school. I don't have a remedy for that. ☺

Chapter 9

Ear Aches and Infections

In the preface to this book, I mentioned the beginning of my journey to seeking for alternatives in healing. The antibiotics my infant son was taking were not working for his ear infections. As I said earlier, I was speaking with a close friend about my second son getting an ear infection and not wanting to repeat what happened with my first son. She shared some wisdom with me that I use to this day.

She said to take equal parts vodka and raw apple cider vinegar with the mother (the floating brown stuff) and put it in a bottle with a dropper. Take half a dropper and warm it and then drop a few drops in the infected ear. Get a hot, wet washcloth and with one hand hold it over the ear. With the other hand massage the muscles from under their armpit down the side of the ribs. What?? That's just weird! Well, I tried it and I'm so glad I did!

I was so nervous driving up to the drive- through liquor store (funny…you're not supposed to drink and drive right?). I had never touched the stuff and I was going to warm it and put it in my son's ear?

I drove up to the window and half hiding my face said, "Can I have one of those little tiny vodka bottles?"

The cashier said in a cheerful voice, "Oh, you mean a spritzer?"

"Uh, yeah I guess." I said nodding my head thinking "What am I doing?"

Well, I mixed it with the apple cider vinegar. I filled the dropper half full and put it in a spoon and put it over the stove. It took only a few seconds for it to get warm enough to put in his ear. It needs to be a little above body temperature but not too hot because you don't want to burn them. I won't lie to you and tell you that he loved it. No one wants anything inside their ear, especially when it is already in extreme pain. So he cried and wiggled, but I needed to keep it in his ear for at least ten minutes and rub down his side.

I learned later that the vodka numbs the ache and both the vinegar and vodka kill the bacteria. The rubbing from the armpit down the side helps to drain the infection. I typically only have to do this once or twice. Seldom have I had to do it more than four times and the infection is gone.

When my kids would cry louder about ten minutes into the treatment my husband was worried that it hurt them because alcohol burns in open wounds. I told him it was fine and that it didn't burn. Well, not too long after that I was able to prove it to him. I got an ear infection and it was killer! I got some ready for myself and put it in my ear, placed the folded hot washcloth over my ear and rubbed down my side. Within about ten minutes my ear started draining and the pressure released. But it was REALLY loud as it popped and gurgled with the pressure release. That's why they were crying. My ear felt plugged for about a week, but the pain was gone. It was worth it.

There is only time that the vodka/vinegar treatment didn't work. I tried at least two treatments a day for about three days and my third son was still hurting. I thought, "Maybe it isn't bacterial, maybe it is viral". I gave him some chaparral tincture and within a day it was gone and he was happy.

My daughter has several times told me that her ear hurts and wants me to put that "stinky stuff" in her ear. I'll give her a treatment and within minutes she takes a nap and when she wakes up it is gone.

As I said in Chapter 2, since we have been off of uncultured cow's milk (fresh store-bought or raw milk), we have not seen an ear infection. Just sayin'....

Chapter 10

The Boo-Boo

When you're dealing with children, you are exposed to all kinds of "owies" and "boo-boos". Everything from burns to scrapes and dings. When you know what to do, there is little stress.

The Open Wound

A few years ago my daughter was skipping along on a sidewalk and within a split second somehow she got the top of her toe stuck under the front part of the sandal and made a "toe sandwich" with the concrete. That little action filleted the top of her little toe. I had recently been to a class that taught the many uses of raw unpasteurized honey. So, I thought I'd give it a try.

This is what I did with the open wound. I did not wash it. I used the honey as a poultice. I got a paper towel and put about two teaspoons of **honey** on it. I wrapped it over the toe, and then to keep the mess to a minimum, wrapped it with a grocery bag. Then I wrapped the whole mess in an Ace- type bandage. I changed it twice a day for two days. An amazing thing happened- a grey matter started to take the place of where the skin used to be. That was brand spakin' new skin growing!! That toe should have scarred, but it didn't.

If the injury is really deep and needs stitches, then it is best to seek medical help. If it is minor and I am not sure how to get the bleeding to stop, I will have capsules of cayenne ready for such an occasion. Cayenne can be sprinkled directly on the bleeding wound and will assist coagulation, but will burn like a crazy horse, so just be ready for that. I have used cayenne also for friends whose periods wouldn't stop for weeks on end (Note: the cayenne was taken internally with capsules not topically applied, yeowsers!) Cayenne is an amazing herb. If stitches are required, I would still put honey on it, because it will help to minimize scarring.

The Burn

One time my second son was riding dad's dirt bike with him. He hopped off and on the way down his little leg landed on the exhaust pipe. We had a second degree burn within seconds. He was screaming in pain. I tried honey directly on the burn, but it was way too painful. So I said a little prayer and went to work. I got a little condiment cup and put about one table spoon of aloe vera, two table spoons of raw honey and a few drops of lavender essential oil and mixed it well. The aloe vera was nice and cool from being in the fridge. I put part of the concoction on a paper towel and applied the goopy mess to his burn. I wrapped it in a grocery bag and then finished it up with an Ace bandage. He calmed down quickly and took a nap. I wrapped it once more that day and then two more times the next day. The third day he said it didn't hurt at all. It looked a whole lot better too.

I did the same thing for my 18- month old niece who burned her fingers by touching the pipe on the wood burning stove. The hardest part was that it felt better and she wanted to keep taking the bandage off and eating the honey. Then it wouldn't feel better anymore and she would cry. But we kept at it, and by morning it felt much better. The blisters looked crazy and painful, but they didn't hurt her.

If you ever experience this, be sure to keep the blisters covered because you want to prevent infection if they pop. If they do pop, don't stress, just keep the honey coming because it will heal.

Scratches, Scrapes and Rashes

I went to a class in the middle of the desert a few years ago and I learned how to make salve. For a few years I've been making this salve that is awesome! I recommend it for scratches, scrapes, and rashes. It is easy and inexpensive to make. The recipe is below.

When my father-in-law was about three years old he fell and scraped his knee pretty bad. He didn't tell his mom and it soon became septic and infected. It was painful and it was a long process to fix it. If his mom would have had salve, she could have applied it and it would have never gotten infected.

I have personally used the salve for eczema issues for myself and it was gone in two days. I have also used it for diaper cream. When my kids have scrapes, scratches, dings and other boo-boos they ask for a little salve. It also works well for bug bites and stings.

Ahhh Salve!

- 1 oz comfrey leaf
- 1 oz chaparral leaf
- 1 oz Oregon Grape root
- 1 oz Osha root
- 1 oz calendula petals
- 1 oz mullein leaf
- 12 oz pure olive oil
- 1 oz beeswax (broken up or grated – it melts faster)
- 2 oz Vodka
- 10 drops lavender essential oil (optional)

Powder all of your herbs with a coffee grinder or a blender. Take the herbs that say "root" and put them in a separate bowl and add the vodka. It should be a sludgy consistency. Let it sit for about an hour. The alcohol opens up the root. Put them in a glass bowl. Turn your oven to its lowest possible setting. 170° or lower is best. Do not let it boil. Let the herbs sit in the oil for 10-12 hours (or longer). Layer cheesecloth in a colander that is resting in a bowl that is a bit larger. A little bit at a time, spoon small portions of the herb/oil mix into the cheesecloth. Squeeze as much of the oil out as you can. Toss the expended herbs in the compost pile. Measure your oils again. You should have close to 8oz of infused oil. If necessary, add olive oil to reach 8oz. Over double boiler (or a small pan inside a medium sized pan half way full of water) heat the beeswax. Once all the beeswax is melted, add your herb infused oil. It will look like egg drop soup. When the wax has melted again, add your essential oil. Pour into containers and let sit undisturbed for about one hour. Then it will be ready to use! If it is too hard for your liking, melt the salve again and add a little more oil. If it is too soft for your liking add a little more beeswax until you are satisfied with the consistency.

I also like to put salve in lip balm containers. It makes it a little easier to use. If this recipe seems too complicated, a salve similar to this one is available for purchase. It can be purchased from www.colonialbloom.com

The salve has had success with not only rashes and scrapes and scratches, but also open sores. One example is, a friend of mine came to me and asked my advice for her brother. He is a roper that kept ripping open his hurt finger. He had tried some remedies (including prescription ointments) and yet the finger still wouldn't heal completely. I recommended using the salve. It healed within a few days and he was amazed.

Bentonite Clay

This clay is one of my favorite tools. I purchase it dry and then when I'm ready to use it, I simply add some water to it in my kitchen aid and "let 'er rip"! When it is a consistency you would use for a clay mask, it is ready. I add about ten drops of rosemary and lavender essential oils to it. You can spoon it into a small glass jar or I pipe it in using a disposable frosting bag (it is a little less messy that way). It will keep for several months. If mold begins to grow, it is time to make a new batch.

This clay is magnetic clay. I have seen it pull bruises out, pull infection to the surface, aid acne infections to the surface and pull the itch from mosquito bites.

My first experience with the clay was amazing! My husband was installing an air-conditioning unit in our room when I hear this clang and grunt. When I went to see what had happened he was in so much pain. He had fallen off the support he was standing on and had twisted his ankle pretty good. I laid him on the floor and took a paper towel and slapped a glob of bentonite on his ankle and wrapped it with an Ace bandage. Once I put it on both sides of his ankle. Within a few minutes he said, "This feel's really weird, it is almost like the two sides are trying to draw to each other. Take one side off!" See, magnetic! In a few days, the outer edges beyond the clay began to show bruising. Another trick I learned from a chiropractor was to put hot, wet towels around his ankle and then ice it. That was repeated every fifteen minutes for an hour a day. He was walking the next day with little assistance. It took some time for the pain to completely go away, but he was able to get around and function fairly comfortably.

Here is another application for bentonite clay. My daughter went to visit a neighbor…barefoot. In the morning she was crying. She had stepped on a rock and it had punctured into her foot and festered overnight. So, we put about a teaspoon size clay blob on a paper towel and put it on the infected area. The clay over the next hour or so drew the infection to the surface. When she was in the tub she was able to squeeze out much of the infection. We did one more round of clay for an hour or so. That afternoon we washed the clay off again and let it dry out a bit. When it was dry we put salve on it. The rock worked its way to the surface. We did salve a few more days to make sure that there was no more infection.

Chapter 11

The Cough Cough

There are a few things that can make a mother want to dye her hair bright orange and admit herself to a funny farm. A constant cough that will not go away or that is incredibly phlegmy is one of those things. The temptation to say, "Would you just stop it?" comes to the lips, but you know it isn't their fault.

Sometimes the cough is allergy related. I don't have much experience with these kinds of coughs.

One of the scariest times in my life is the first time one of my children had a rumbly cough that sounded like a seal bark. He could hardly breathe. I feared pneumonia. When we got home from a long trip at one in the morning, I headed to the hospital with my nine month old son. When I got there they told me it was only croup (I should be relieved...right?). They said it was viral and that all I could do was wait. I was instructed to give Tylenol every four hours and alternate it every two hours with Ibuprofen. That seemed like a lot of medicine that wasn't for the cough, but I did it anyway.

I have learned since then that there is something I can do. I would treat the fever like I described in Chapter 7. Recently my third son started croup coughing in the middle of the night. When I got up to help him, I gave him licorice root. By morning the cough had changed from "seal bark" to a normal cough. The reason it sounds like a "seal bark" is because the bronchials are inflamed. Mullein will bring down the inflammation. If it is cold outside, the cool air can also help bring down the inflammation. I continued to give him licorice root (which tastes good and he liked the sweetness) for the next few days. The cough was gone quickly. The huge difference between the first time I dealt with this specific cough and the last time is the healing time. I was only up one night and not every night for a week.

Bronchitis is one of the most annoying conditions to deal with. The constant cough is enough to drive you mad. My oldest had this for weeks and weeks until we got him on an antibiotic. I have recently learned that rosemary essential oil (I put it in a capsule because it can taste bad) can kill bacterial bronchitis and kill the cough. Amazing! It takes a few days and it should be taken for at least three days after the cough is gone so that all the bacteria are gone.

Sometimes coughs accompany bacterial and viral infections. While you're waiting for the infection to clear up, I use a chest rub. I don't get the stuff at the grocery store that is petroleum based. I started making my own. I use white beeswax because it doesn't stain, the yellow one can leave a slight yellow color around the collar of clothes.

Breathey Rub

- 1 oz beeswax (white or yellow)
- 8 oz pure olive oil
- 100 drops eucalyptus essential oil
- 100 drops rosemary essential oil
- 100 drops camphor essential oil
- 100 drops wintergreen essential oil
- 100 drops peppermint essential oil
- 10 oz container

Over a double boiler (or a small pan inside a medium sized pan half way full of water) on medium heat melt the beeswax. Add the olive oil. Continue to heat until the beeswax melts. Remove from heat and add your essential oils. Give it a good stir and then pour it into your container.

Chapter 12

Cold, Flu and Strep

When my children get any strain of a cold or flu it is important to act quickly. The sooner you can get them on the road to healing, the sooner those viruses can die and not embed themselves.

My favorite tincture combination to boost the immune system and fighting power at first sight is awesome.

Kick It Tincture

- .25 oz Chaparral
- .25 oz Goldenseal
- .25 oz Osha root
- .25 Yerba santa
- 5 oz vodka, half vegetable glycerin/ half water or vinegar

Follow the instructions found in Chapter 4. In my family, adults would use two squirts three or four times a day. For our children five to 12, I'd use one squirt three times a day. For smaller children I'd use less than half a squirt. I'd do this for about a week to make sure we were in the clear.

If I didn't catch it in time, I would still use this tincture and follow the instructions for fever and cough in the previous chapters.

Strep

Our family has had many, many bouts with strep. It is not a good idea to just ride it out because it can weaken the heart and lead to rheumatic fever. But I have successfully used goldenseal root and Oregon grape root combo to take care of that problem. I took it for a week three times a day. This makes sure all those little buggers are gone. Some sources say that goldenseal is too strong for small children. If Oregon grape root doesn't kick the strep, I would use only a few drops of goldenseal with the Oregon grape root.

Also, keep in mind that if I continue to get an infection over and over there is a chance my spleen is weak and in need of strengthening. I can take yarrow to strengthen that and also clean the blood. I learned that also with my cold sores. They have been recurring since childhood, and yarrow helped a bunch with continual outbreaks. I took a few squirts of yarrow two to three times a day for a few weeks. The outbreaks are now so few and far between that I hardly remember I had them almost once a month for years.

Chapter 13

To Immunize or Not

Every family has to decide what is right for them. I believe nothing regarding health care can be more controversial than immunizations. With the rise of autism and the fear of it being linked to the mercury- based preservatives, there is no wonder it is a hot topic.

If you look at the other side, I have seen pictures of what diseases like polio and measles do to children. It can be frightening.

I have talked to people in the conventional and alternative medical fields who will not immunize for many different reasons. The scare tactics used to convince you that you need to give your children immunizations (beginning at birth) 36 shots is a little out of control in my opinion.

It is easy to go to YouTube and look up video after video (uploaded by the parent) of children who were normal and developing perfectly until they were given an MMR or DPT shots, and all of the sudden withdrew from socializing, became very ill and back peddled from speech or motor skills. You don't have to be a rocket scientist to see the correlation.

I believe the intentions of Louis Pasteur were pure and well-intentioned when the first immunizations were invented and developed. I do not believe those intentions are still pure by companies who stand to make billions by these "required" immunizations.

When I was questioning if immunizations were right for our family, the more I researched, the angrier I became. I prayed about it. My answer was, "Do not be so judgmental." I didn't quite understand. However; I made my decision. Until I found a safer alternative, I would abstain from these inoculations.

There is a website called vaers.hhs.gov (Vaccine Adverse Event Reporting System) that may interest some readers. If a doctor chooses to report a vaccine injury, they can. The numbers can be astounding. In 2004 the number of babies that died from the actual Hepatitis B disease were in the twenties. The babies who died from the shot were over 1,200. Those numbers aren't very good. Those numbers also don't show an accurate number because these are merely the doctors who *chose* to report the injury.

Some families wait until the child is just about to enter school before they get their shots. I think that is a good compromise if parents feel uneasy about it giving shots to a baby, yet still worry about these diseases.

The big problem I have with the whole vaccine "thing" is that the only "trusted" information comes from the people who make it. They also happen to be the ones who stand to make lots and lots of money preying on the fear of people who trust them wholeheartedly.

I have recently learned of a little thing called "nosodes" that are homeopathic medications. Nosodes are used all around the world. I have read reports of nosodes being used successfully in Cuba and France for outbreaks of different diseases. These are extremely inexpensive to make and there are no side effects because the doses are so small, yet effective. Information on these remedies is somewhat suppressed in the United States. However, homeopathic doctors can prescribe them. There is also a website called www.elixirs.com where you can purchase what you desire for your family's protection.

When we are self-reliant in any field, to understand principles-that is when the fear recedes. Then we have the tools we need.

Use your own judgment. Let the Spirit guide you. Yours might be a different direction than mine.

Chapter 14

Sources

In this chapter I will give many of the sources that I have used. Hopefully they will be of great use to you as you continue learning of ways to become self-reliant with the health care of your family.

Books:

Ancient Natural Remedies by Peter Bigfoot (www.revismountain.org)

Modern Essentials Usage Guide (www.aromatools.com)

Herbs:

www.mountainroseherbs.com

Essential Oils:

http://www.doterra.myvoffice.com/marshalpetitt/

http://www.mountainroseherbs.com/aroma/ess.html

How to Use Essential Oils:

www.everythingessential.me

Premade Concoctions

www.colonialbloom.com

www.reevismountain.org

Containers: (dark glass jars, tins and beeswax for salves)
www.mountainroseherbs.com

www.ingramcontent.com/pod-product-compliance
Lightning Source LLC
Chambersburg PA
CBHW070342290526
45791CB00003B/1434